WHY YOU SHOULD AVOID SEDENTARY LIFESTYLE!

Always remember "Health is Wealth"

Table of Contents

CHAPTER ONE

SEDENTARY LIFESTYLE

It is a lifestyle in which one sits or lies down a lot with very little or no exercise at all. It is also called "Inactive lifestyle".

Wikipedia defined it as a lifestyle type characterized by an abundance of sedentary behaviours. This lifestyle has increased drastically over few decades due to an increase in office jobs that requires sitting down. It also increases due to the fact that so many do not know the therapeutic effect of exercise.

Majority do not exercise at this present time. Many people are so much dependent on other means of transportation order than through walking, even when the distance is obviously close-by.

-If you are often sitting or lying down when carrying out some activities such as; Using a mobile phone, playing video game, reading newspaper or other books, chatting with friends on social media, watching television or operating your PC.

-If you do not have time for exercise. You just walk from your house to your car, to your office (sitting one place often), from your office back to your house. It is an indication of a sedentary lifestyle.

Sedentary lifestyle brings about the following life-threatening conditions:

-Cardiovascular disease

-Lipid disorder

-Diabetes

-Obesity

-Cancer

-Osteoporosis

-Depression

-Anxiety

-Vein-related problems

Cardiovascular disease

Not getting enough exercise can cause heart disease. This can include coronary heart disease which can lead to myocardial infarction or cardiomyopathy which alters the way your heart pumps blood.

Some other things can bring about cardiovascular diseases but sedentary lifestyle is a high contributing factor.

Being less active puts one at a higher risk of developing high blood pressure.

Not being active gives rise to the deposition of fatty plaques along the walls of arteries, which can finally lead to heart attack or stroke.

Lipid disorder

Cholesterol is a fat-like substance that body needs to build healthy cells. A good cholesterol is referred to as high density lipoprotein (HDL), which helps to get rid of the bad cholesterol (LDL) from the bloodstream. When you do not exercise enough, you may have high LDL while you have HDL that is not enough, which can lead to hardening of arteries and other vascular issues.

Diabetes

The hormone in the body that helps it use sugar for energy, is called insulin. Living an inactive or sedentary lifestyle for a long-time can result in changes in your body which may cause insulin resistance which gives rise to Type 2 diabetes.

Type 2 diabetes is commonly diagnosed in adults but children can also develop it. Juvenile or Type 1 diabetes is commonly seen in children.

Obesity

Sedentary lifestyle indicates that there is less movement. When movement is less, calories burned are also less, which results in accumulation of body fat leading to weight gain and in the long run causes obesity. Sedentary lifestyle is supportive of all causes of mortality, of which obesity is one of them. Regular exercise and diet control reduce excess fat from the body. As aerobic exercise also improves the cardiorespiratory fitness, resistance training also strengthens muscles.

Cancer

Inactive lifestyle gives room for the development of cancers. Being more physically active and taking healthy diets reduce your risk of developing cancer. Some studies show that the amount of time people spend in seated position is in relationship with a higher possibility of death from cancer.

Osteoporosis

Sedentary behaviours cause decrease in bones which makes the bones fragile, brittle, and weak, placing them at high risk of getting fractured easily.

Why osteoporosis is very dangerous is that it progresses silently without any noticeable symptoms. It always remains silent until the bone fractures.

Depression

Leading a sedentary lifestyle gives rise to depression. Happy hormones released in the brain through physical activity are dopamine and serotonin. They are very helpful to us in maintaining mood balance which provides us with positive feelings and motivation.

When leading a sedentary lifestyle, they are not being released and thus giving rise to depression.

Sedentarism also gives rise to anxiety and some other mental illnesses. Some previous studies on the repercussions of sedentary behaviour, linked excessive sitting with health problems.

Vein-related problems

During sedentarism, calf muscles are not doing their job and venous blood flow slows down. It is the work of the calf-muscles to contract there-by propelling the venous blood from your feet and leg back to the heart during physical activity.

When the action of the calf muscles is no longer there, there is a higher possibility of a thrombus forming in the veins, like the popliteal vein.

When a thrombus is formed in a deep vein, it is referred to as deep venous thrombosis (DVT), but if it occurs in a superficial vein, it is referred to as superficial venous thrombosis (SVT). Slow blood flow resulting from sedentarism also leads to varicosity and spider veins. It also leads to swelling of bilateral feet and leg. Legs and feet swelling are always observed by some students during exam period, when they always sit one place for a long-time reading and revising.

When a thrombus dislodges, it is referred to as an embolus. When this embolus gets to a smaller blood vessel, especially arteries, it blocks blood flow there by restricting oxygen supply to that area. If it occurs in the brain, it causes cerebrovascular accident, popularly known as stroke (in this case specifically referred to as ischemic stroke).

Embolus can get to the lungs and cause pulmonary embolism or to the heart and cause coronary heart disease which gives rise to angina and myocardial infarction.

CHAPTER TWO

How to stop or avoid sedentarism

-Do not go by your car often:

The means through which we travel in the modern age is associated with rates of overweight and obesity. Active modes such as walking or cycling have a lot of health benefits and prevents the diseases or disorders associated with sedentary lifestyle.

Taking public transit even lowers BMI more than going in your own car. You have to walk to the park and also climb the steps of the bus. All these are physical activities which are graded higher compared to those ones you experience when taking your personal car.

Get a treadmill and/or cycle ergometer you will be using for exercise in your house at any time you wish, especially before and after going to work. You can even keep some in the office, for you to use during break. Having dumbbells and exercise rope, will also be awesome.

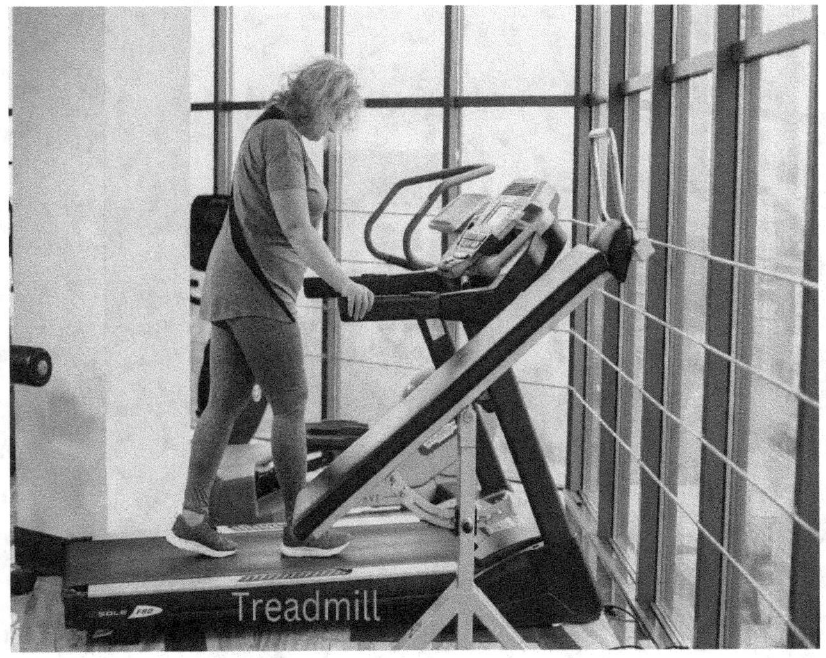

Fig 2.0 Treadmill

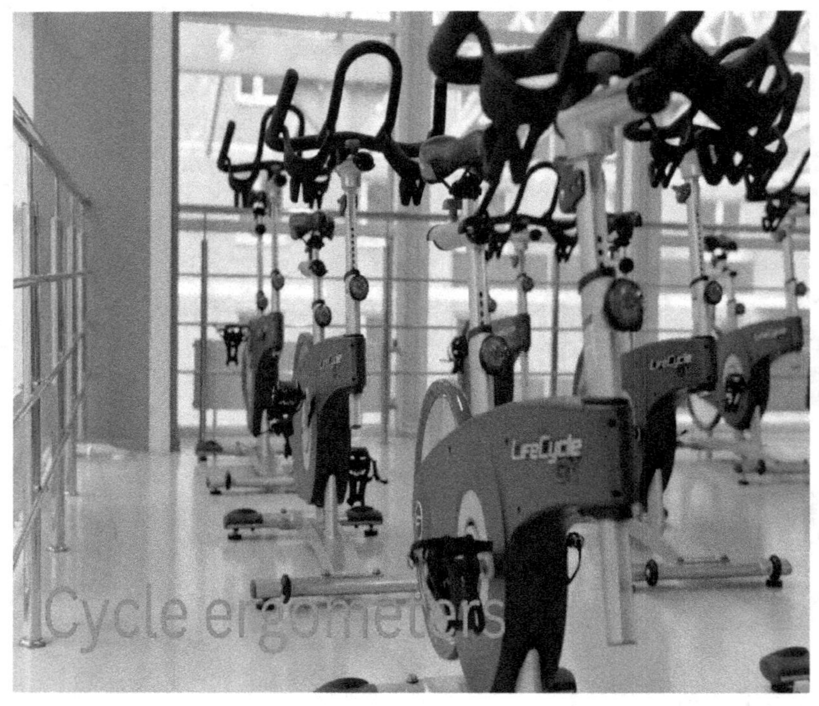

Fi

g 2.1 Cycle ergometer

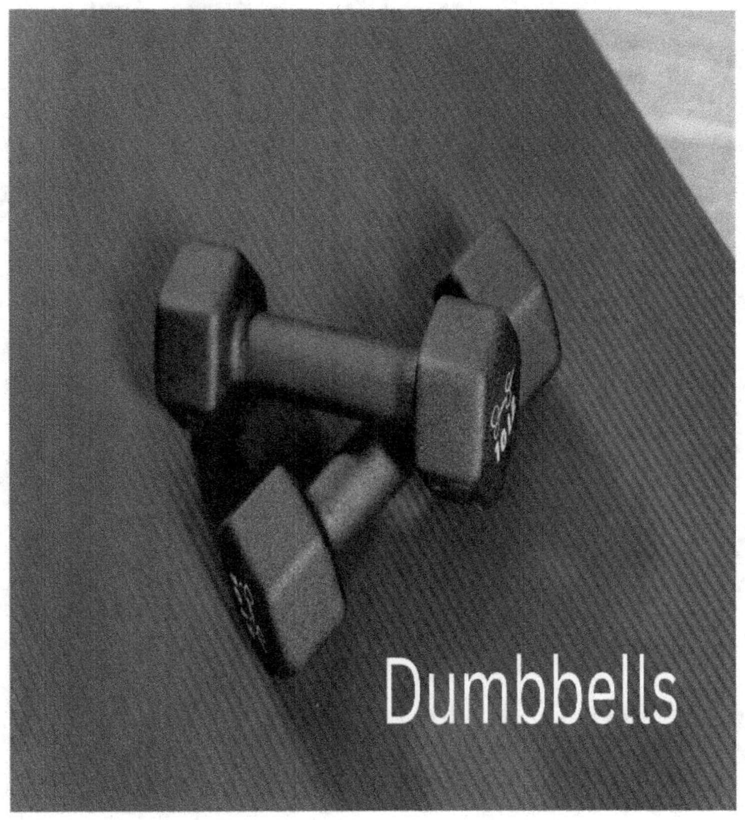

Fig 2.2 Dumbbells

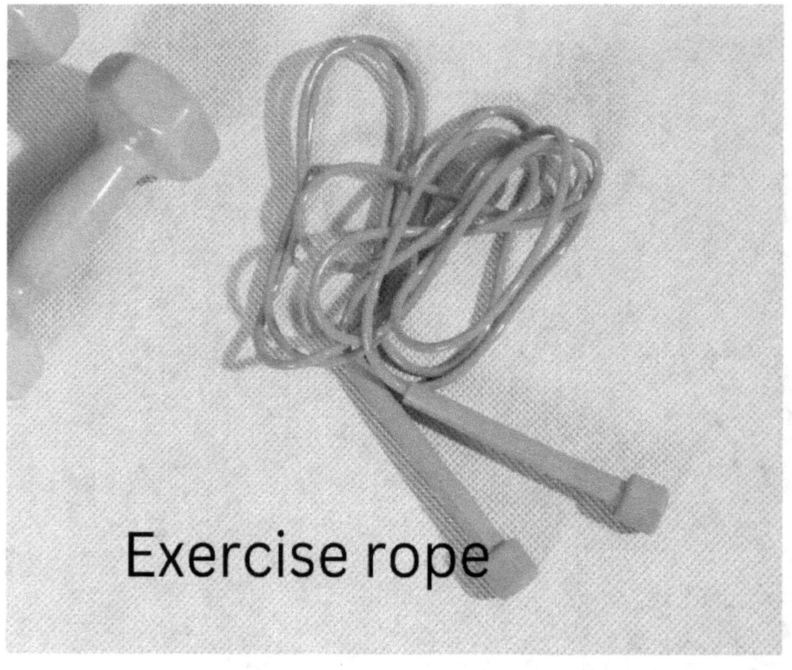

Fig 2.3 Exercise rope

-Carry out your chores:

Instead of moving from table to the bed after eating, sweep and clean your environment and arrange your house. Sweeping keeps the body very active.

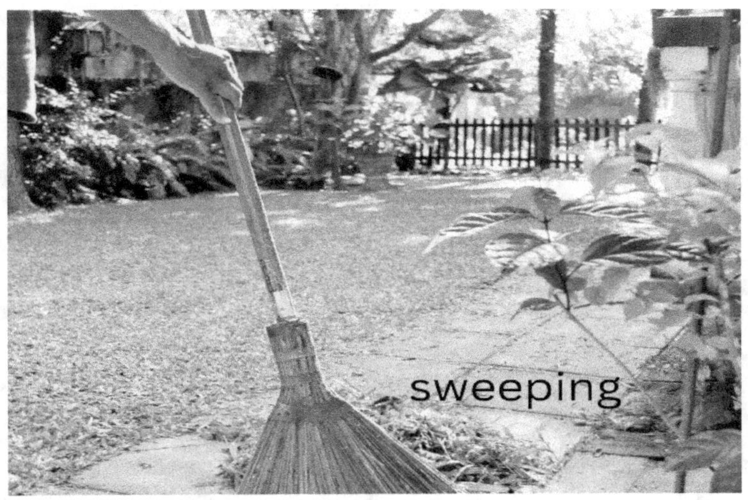

Fig 2.4 Sweeping

If you don't want to go out to run, you can go with the options of buying a treadmill or bicycle ergometer as I earlier suggested, so that you can now exercise within the comfort of your room or house.

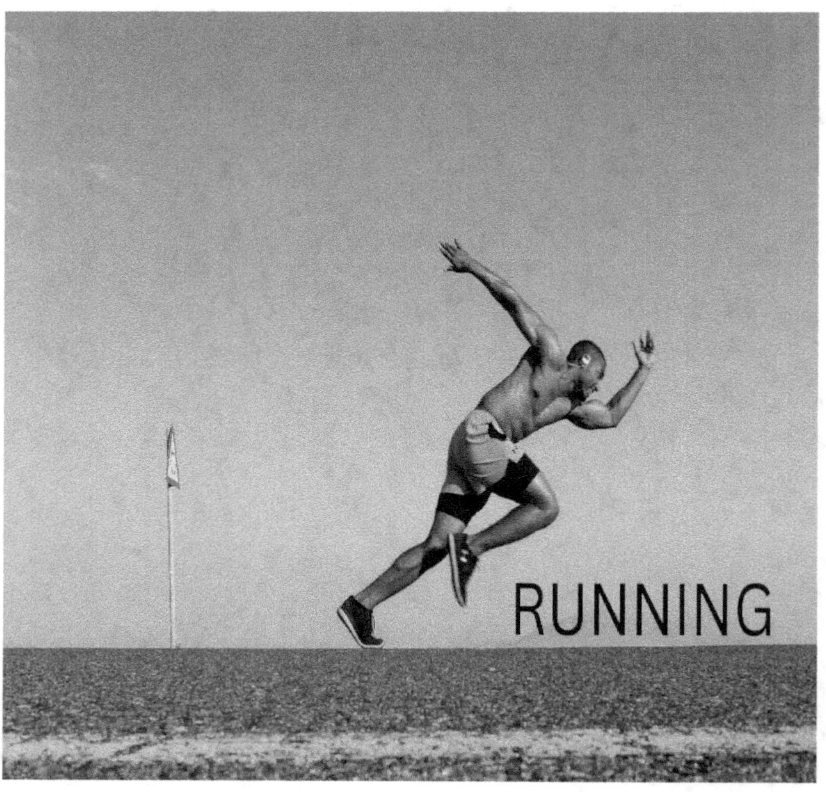

Fig 2.5 Running

Always remember that exercise has progressions. If you want to start newly, do not just start with vigorous activities. It will also be pretty good if you let your healthcare provider know that you want to start your exercise if you have any underlying condition(s).

-At work, always get up and move around:

After 30mins, get up and stroll around your working place. You can just take a walk to a co-worker's desk instead of sending e mail. Always try your best to perform activities while strolling such as answering calls instead of sitting whenever feasible.

-Always practice active ankle pump exercises: Whenever you are seated, always try and move your feet up and down continuously. It enhances venous return. The movement should only occur in the ankle joints.

-Running errands:

It's something good and great turning errand to work out by going from errand to errand by walking.

CHAPTER THREE

Recommendations:

For individuals that are disabled, such as stroke patients, spinal cord injury patients, osteoarthritic patients, patients with Parkinson's disease, patients with spondylosis, etcetera, should have a physiotherapist that gives them treatments. The physiotherapist will help to make sure you avoid sedentary lifestyle and help in keeping your body fit.

Summary

Always remember the saying, that "health is wealth". Do what can improve your health and avoid those associated with health risks. Endeavor to live an active lifestyle and avoid those life-threatening conditions discussed above. Keep living healthy and enjoying. Thanks a lot!

www.ingramcontent.com/pod-product-compliance
Lightning Source LLC
Chambersburg PA
CBHW051729250726
48653CB00008B/3277